The Eight Principles of Good Health

Modern Health Advice from an Ancient Healing System

EzDean Fassassi

DEDICATION

Exclusively pursuing physical wellness
Is a fruitless endeavor
Lest one also seek
to cultivate a loving heart

To all those in pursuit of *holistic* wellbeing...

CONTENTS

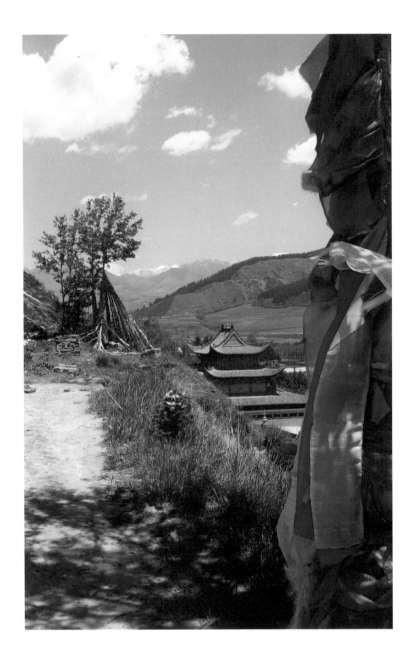

A view from Serkhog Valley, historical Eastern Amdo Tibet

ACKNOWLEDGMENTS

Years of struggling to explain the practical applications of Tibetan Medical Science to friends, family, and patients has ultimately led to the writing of this book. Should there be any merit in this work, I am indebted to those around me who have urged the distillation of these understandings in a concise and accessible format. A special thanks to my family, especially my wife Amber for her support, and sister Bilqis Fassassi who played a large role in editing the very first drafts. And finally, to all of my teachers, mentors, and guides: I am eternally grateful.

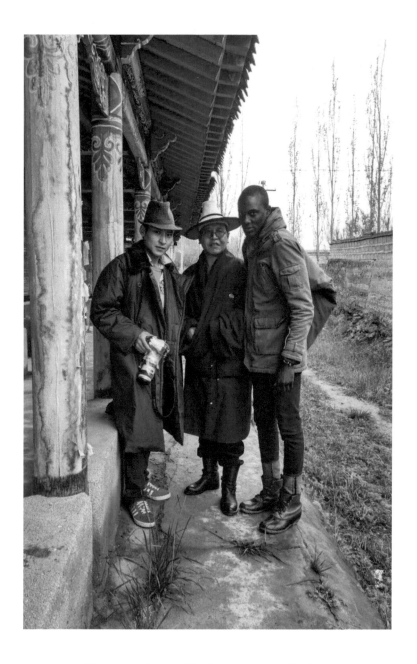

The author with two friends at a monastery in Amdo

PREFACE

The Second Edition of The Eight Principles of Good Health was inspired by art, beauty, memories, naturescapes, and visual aesthetics, on the whole. Since my first foray into Western China or historical Eastern Amdo Tibet in 2009, there have been the most vivid images scored into my mind's eye. Although I took very few photos, I somehow managed to scrounge up enough of a collection enabling me to faithfully depict the various themes of this manual.

My experience in studying this beautiful healing system was at times painful and tedious, but ultimately very rewarding. The lessons learned were not isolated to the classroom or clinic, rather, my entire living experience in that part of the world was pervaded by a didactic energy, seemingly fine-tuned to instruct every aspect of this sacred medical science. At times I was learning about the proper conduct of the physician; at other times I would observe the manifest symptomology of both physiological and psychological disorders, yet my favorite was in observing the parallels of the human condition, in nature. As stated in the teaching: "As without, so within." The faces, landscapes, meals, and other full-color photos in this Second Edition are an attempt to share the beauty of my experience in pursuing this teaching, which ultimately lead to the writing of this book. Should these personal photos convey even a little part of this ineffable sentiment, then it was well worth the revision.

I would be remiss if I did not acknowledge the artistic inspiration of my friend, and accomplished Tibetan photographer Tsemdo Thar, whose work has inspired me for many years. Through these visual aids, the intent is for this manual of healing to become even more vibrant and accessible to a general audience.

EzDean Fassassi

November 2019
Gaithersburg, MD

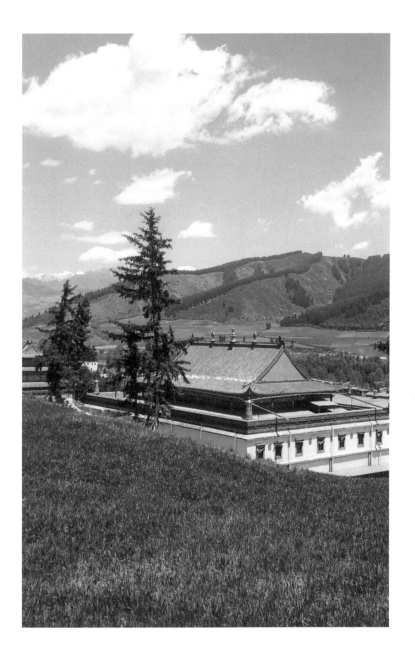

Serkhog Monastery, Amdo

INTRODUCTION

If you're reading this, it's likely that you're interested in the subject of how to maintain or restore proper health, either for yourself or someone that you care about. You probably don't care that I'm not a medical doctor, or that Tibetan Medical Science is something you're scarcely familiar with. It is with all of that in mind that I will endeavor to make this as informative, yet concise as possible.

Tibetan Medical Science—as I like to call it—is a centuries-old system of healing that is even more relevant today. In the mire that is the surfeit of legitimate but uncontextualized health advice and questionable nutritionist doctrines, this medical system offers an elegant, simple, yet profoundly effective explanatory model for understanding what health and disease really are. This "Science of Healing," as it is colloquially referred to, is inherently holistic, as it deals with any and every disease and considers the various parts and systems of the body to be intimately connected. To perceive the connectedness of the body's various systems is the hallmark of medical holism; furthermore, to perceive the connection between the individual and the environment, in which said individual exists, is consistent, thorough, and responsible medicine.

Although the 5900 verses of the Tibetan medical canon, literally translated as "The Secret Tantra of Quintessential Instructions on The Eight Branches of Deathlessness," have been preserved in the Tibetan language, it is a healing system for all of humanity. This teaching is not restricted to any ethnicity, nationality, or creed, though it is unapologetically couched in Tibetan culture and a Buddhist worldview.

The therapeutic interventions in Tibetan Medical Science, or its methods of healing, are categorized into four distinct levels, in descending order of importance and effectiveness:

1. Diet
2. Lifestyle
3. Medicines
4. Accessory Therapies

I would like to briefly elaborate on each of these levels in order to demonstrate that Diet is the most essential and effective method of healing. A proper diet is not just for prevention, but Tibetan Medical Science asserts that Diet is principal in re-establishing health in a diseased body. Therefore, any disease must be treated, at least in part, through a wholesome diet.

Lifestyle is second on the list. This describes one's behavior and daily habits: how one sleeps, works, eats, dresses, sits, exercises, *et cetera*.

The third level of therapy is Medicines. They have a more rapid, albeit shallow effect than Diet or Lifestyle modifications. Furthermore, because it may be more difficult for some to change their dietary or lifestyle habits than it would be to take a pill, potion, or injection, medicines may thus be regarded as being a more convenient and straightforward option for helping redress imbalance—necessitating little to no change on behalf of the patient, perhaps other than to remember to take the medicine at regularly prescribed times.

Lastly, on the fourth and final level of therapeutic intervention in Tibetan Medical Science, we have Accessory Therapies. Although the interventions on this level create an effect that is even more rapidly perceived than that of Medicines, therapies such as massage, cupping, energy healings, acupuncture, surgery, and the like, are generally less effective at purging the root cause of illness. For instance, a recurring dietary allergy or a persistent lower back pain cannot solely be addressed by acupuncture—Diet and Lifestyle modifications are paramount, else treatment will eventually, over time, prove ineffective. Nevertheless, in some instances, a very "shallow" (non-deeply-rooted) disorder can exclusively be cleared away by Medicines or Accessory Therapies. Examples of such etiologies are bio-physical traumas, like muscle aches and pains caused by a recent accident, or a case of poisoning from food, alcohol or venom. In Tibetan Medical Science, such ailments are said to be "near causes" of disease and can readily be alleviated by Medicines or Accessory Therapies, alone. Excepting such etiologies, without the proper Diet and Lifestyle modifications to re-establish and maintain the healthy state, the effect of the aforementioned therapies will be short-lived.

To reiterate, the list above is numbered in descending order of therapeutic importance and effectiveness. This means that Medicines are only the third-most essential and effective of the therapeutic interventions, which is counter to what most people believe. Therefore, no matter how expensive or effective a pill, be it prescribed by a Western medical doctor, or an alternative health-care professional, Diet and Lifestyle remain more essential and effective for the overall re-establishment of the patient's health than Medicines. In the same way, an Accessory Therapy, such as a highly effective surgical procedure performed with cutting-edge technology, or even an energy healing by a spiritually inclined practitioner, is not as essential or effective to the re-establishment of overall health, as Diet and Lifestyle modifications. Again, the exception is that relatively simple, non-deeply-rooted issues can be remedied entirely with Medicines or Accessory Therapies alone. However, for anything else, Medicines and Accessory Therapies must invariably be accompanied by Diet and Lifestyle modifications, or their overall therapeutic effect will be minimal.

At this point, some readers may be wondering: "If this is true, why then is there such an emphasis on using Medicines (pills, powders, tinctures, syrups, injections, etc.) in a variety of medical systems, be it modern conventional medicine, or even in many alternative and complementary medical practices?" The answer is complex. The very word "medicine" is literally indistinguishable from the topic, as it tends to be employed as the synecdochal referent to entire healing systems. Books can, and should be written on this linguistic, anthropological, sociological and economic phenomenon. Here, it will only be said that the modern reductionist view of medicine is largely driven by economic interests, though in the past, it may have simply been a result of an inability to reconcile medical breakthroughs made during the European Enlightenment, and previous medical knowledge. The success of 18th and 19th-century developments in medicine contributed to an overreliance on medicines, which persists to this day. Advancements in the study of Infectious Diseases made possible by the invention of the microscope, ultimately led to the development of Germ Theory. The effect was immediately perceptible to all, as death rates from sepsis, infection, and poor hygiene plummeted, and countless lives were saved as a result. Over time, the traditional physician-healer's potions, powders, and exotic implements were fetishized. This was largely due to the public's poor understanding of the science behind the medicine. Resultingly, the effects of these new medical practices were nothing short of magical. It is in this context that the more mundane aspects of medical therapies, in Diet and Lifestyle, may have very likely taken a back seat.

At the time of this writing, the majority of the world's population no longer suffers from infectious diseases, rather, increasingly high rates of morbidity and mortality are assigned to what has been dubbed, "lifestyle" (*viz.* Diet and Lifestyle) diseases. *The Eight Principles of Good Health*, aspires to address this pandemic by re-introducing the ancient wisdom of Tibetan Medical Science, which establishes the preeminence of Diet and Lifestyle therapies, by way of systematic and scientific—albeit non-Western—exposition.

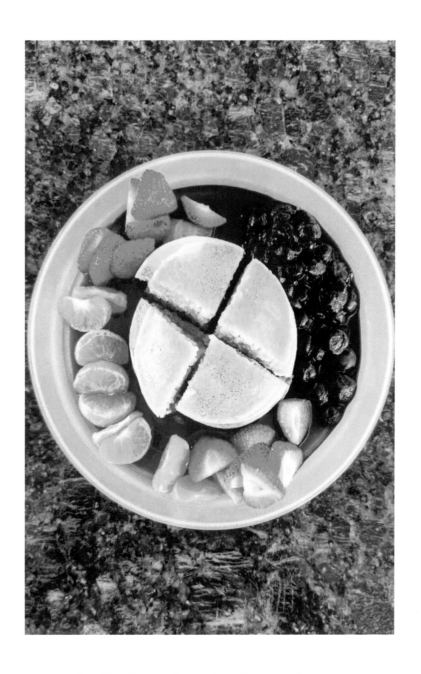

*Breakfast: Buttermilk pancakes with organic clementines,
strawberries, blueberries, and maple syrup*

1 PORTION SIZE

The human stomach is approximately the size of one's fist. Although it can expand considerably, from an anatomical perspective, it isn't all that big.

The canon of Tibetan Medical Science states that were it divided into four, the stomach, at any given time should only be filled up with one-part food and two-parts liquid, leaving one-part empty for digestion. This practice, alone, significantly promotes overall health by helping prevent indigestion. Frequently overeating, from the perspective of Tibetan Medical Science, weakens the effect of the *digestive heat*, which leads to what is commonly referred to as "slow metabolism."[1] This occurs in the following way: frequent overeating overwhelms the stomach's digestive capabilities, as there is insufficient heat energy to process the excess food matter introduced into it. The undigested food matter—consisting of both nutriment and waste product—accumulates in the stomach, creating a dense mucus-like layer around the stomach's walls as well as in the *channels* leading out of the stomach.[2] This creates

---

[1] The "digestive heat" is a literal translation of a very important concept in Tibetan Medical Science. It can be likened to the cooking flame under a cauldron, if that cauldron were the stomach.

[2] In Tibetan Medical Science, the term "channels" refers to the plurality of conduits of conveyance in our bodies, be they nerves, blood, lymphatic vessels, or channels of the non-gross (non-visible) anatomy. In this

additional issues in assimilation and elimination, as the undigested food matter creates blockages for the transference of digested nutriment elsewhere in the body, as well as for waste products, out of the body. It is therefore understandable why indigestion is considered to be "the mother of all diseases" in Tibetan Medical Science.

To further illustrate the importance of proper digestion, please consider that all of the body's primary constituent materials, in addition to their by-products, are direct results of digestive processes. According to Tibetan Medical Science, any food introduced into the system is said to take an average of six days to fully digest and assimilate. The very first by-product of any food substance is an acidic mucous-like substance. The nutriment of that food then passes through nine channels to the liver, and blood is produced—the by-product of which is bile. On the second day, the refined aspect of the blood produces muscle tissue and a by-product of phlegm, saliva, and sweat. The third day fats are produced, with a by-product of body oils. On the fourth day of digestion and assimilation, bone is produced with a by-product of hair, teeth and nails. On the fifth day, bone marrow is produced with a by-product of oily stool. Finally, on the sixth day *dang* is produced with a by-product of the body's reproductive fluids.[3]

Symptoms of slowed or weak metabolism are frequent belching, flatulence, pain in the stomach after eating and, or, shortly after waking from slumber, and heavy mucus production throughout the sinuses.

---

instance we are specifically referring to the nine channels connecting the stomach to the liver, through which the refined products of stomach digestion traverse to make blood and bile.

[3] "Dang" is the ultimate product of digestion, so much so, that its by-product is the body's reproductive fluids! There are no analogues for it in Western biomedicine. It is responsible for an individual's splendor and vitality. It is the ineffable "presence" of a magnanimous being. A physical substance that can be found in the heart, its effect reaches the entire body. Persons deficient in *dang* will experience excessive amounts of fear, depression, weakness and will present as physically feeble.

The best way to achieve the recommended portion size is to begin by being mindful of the intention to eat the recommended portion size—perhaps even visualizing it, and then trusting one's body-intelligence to follow through. The Tibetan medical canon also states that if the recommendation on portion size is correctly adhered to, an individual should be able to do light exercise without much discomfort, immediately after finishing a meal.

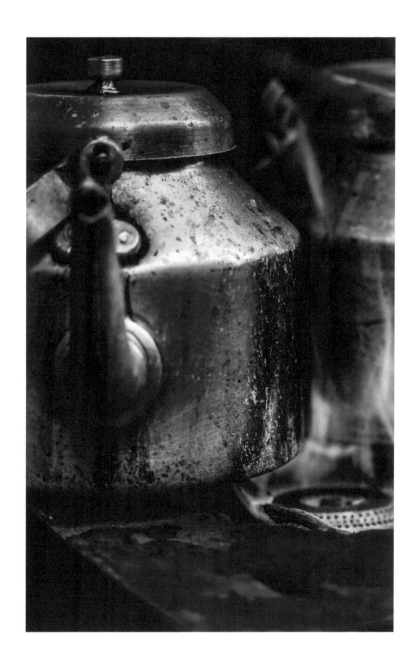

Hot water kettle over a gas stove: Water boiled within 24 hours
is a panacea with no contraindication

2 WATER INTAKE

As carbon-based lifeforms, water is an essential part of our constitution. In fact, the human infant body can be made of up to 75% water, while a full-sized adult will be made of a little less: 55-65%. Either way, water accounts for more than half of the human body's total volume, and as such, is essential to its proper psychological and physiological functioning.

How much water should one consume daily? Believe it or not, the adage of eight US cups is consistent with the general principles of water intake in Tibetan Medical Science. It is, however, important to note that this daily recommendation also includes fluids from other sources, such as non-water drinks, and even food. While that may be true, there is simply no substitute for plain water, which must prominently feature in any balanced diet. Carbonated club soda, flavored water, light tea, soup, and other such fluids should not be regarded as equivalents. Individuals who smoke, regularly consume diuretic beverages (like coffee, soda, or strong black tea), are pregnant, or perspire profusely through disease or strenuous exercise, will need more water than average.

Although bottled water is commonly viewed as the ideal source for fresh, quality water, it is important to consider that many companies use thin and inexpensive plastics as receptacles, and that these containers are typically transported long distances in non-climate-controlled vehicles, only to be stored for indeterminate periods of time before being sold to the consumer. There is, therefore, a high probability that the non-inert substances that these water bottles are made of may leach into the water that they contain, ultimately contaminating the beverage.

Ideally, one should consume fresh water that has not been stagnant in any way. If not from a clean natural source such as rainwater, well water, or river water, then boiling water through which no gross impurity is perceptible will yield pure water—and it will remain so for up to 24 hours. In Tibetan Medical Science, any water which has been stagnant for more than 24 hours is considered stale and should ideally be re-purified before consumption.

Boiling clear water does not just yield potable drink. In Tibetan Medical Science, freshly boiled water is regarded as a panacea with no contraindication. Even when cooled, it has a "light" quality to it; and when consumed hot, freshly-boiled water promotes internal warming, relief from all "cold-natured disorders," and lightness of body.[4] Left to cool, this water can also be consumed by patients with "hot-natured disorders" and with no contraindication.[5]

In sum, everyone, without exception, should regularly consume water. In most cases, this water should at least be room temperature, as this is less shocking to the system given that it is closer to the internal body temperature. Best practice is to regularly

---

[4] In Tibetan Medical Science, what characterizes a disorder as either "cold" or "hot" has little to do with temperature. Rather, what is being referred to is an existential quality. I purposefully use the word "existential" as these properties are derived from the 5 Elements of phenomenology in Tibetan Buddhist cosmology (see p.16 for a brief discussion on the 5 Elements). So-called "cold-natured disorders" can include anything from upper-respiratory issues, obesity, indigestion, belching, nausea, constipation, chronic fatigue, migraines, polyuria, hiccups, and much more.

[5] So-called "hot-natured disorders" are represented by fevers, sharp intestinal pains, chronic body odor, diarrhea, infectious diseases of all kinds, skin irritations, and the like.

consume freshly boiled water, for the reasons stated above. Americans, however, seem to be fond of ice water. This should be consumed in moderation, and ideally limited to the following circumstances: when in warmer climes; when the body's temperature is high, as when engaged in strenuous exercise; when excessively feverish; and lastly, when consuming very spicy, salty or sour foods. Furthermore, water should be consumed in accordance with the body's needs, and not forced upon the system to meet a certain quota. It should seldom, if ever, be consumed in large amounts in short periods of time; rather, best practice is to gradually drink small amounts of water throughout the day—in and around meal times—focusing mostly on when the body's thirst response is triggered.

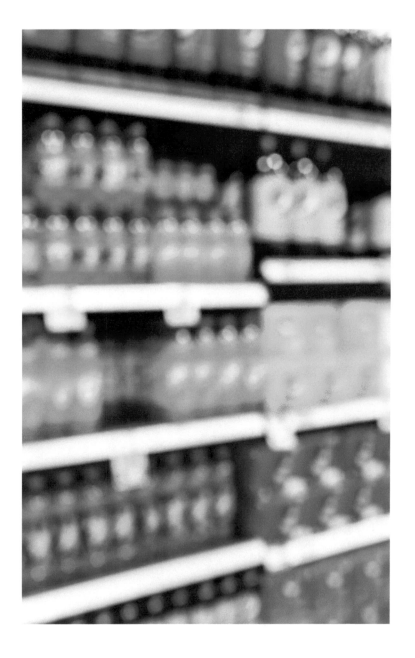

The soft drinks aisle at a U.S. supermarket:
A haven for High Fructose Corn Syrup

3 AVOIDING FAKE FOOD

Over-processed foods are at the root of the epidemic of so-called "lifestyle diseases." Heart disease, stroke, obesity, Type 2 diabetes, etc., have taken over from infectious diseases as the most lethal threats to life in the U.S. Unfortunately, many people still don't know the difference between sugar and High Fructose Corn Syrup—its ubiquitous, less expensive, and more harmful step-cousin. While both are sweet in taste, the former is natural, while the latter is synthetic.

Though a glance at the nutrition facts label on the average packaged foodstuff will reveal a bevy of synthetic ingredients, in my experience, the most injurious of them all is the aforementioned High Fructose Corn Syrup. This sweetener is used in everything from bread, breakfast cereals, ketchup and pickles to mayonnaise, pasta sauces, and soft drinks.

From the perspective of Tibetan Medical Science, High Fructose Corn Syrup and other synthetic ingredients are considered poisons, as, by definition, they are not readily recognized by the human body, and initially trigger an antigenic response. Consequently, these ingredients and the food that is made with them are slow to metabolize, assimilate, and ultimately be evacuated from the system. In plain terms, such substances gradually contribute to the blockage of channels in the body, leading to excess mucus production, chronic indigestion, and the morass of diseases that those issues can engender.

As there are many non-natural ingredients in our modern foodstuffs, it is not always possible to avoid every single one. However, a useful technique is to pay attention to the nature of the foremost ingredients when reading nutrition labels. Food labels, worldwide, respect the same convention of having ingredients present in greatest quantity listed first. Therefore, if a non-natural ingredient is one of the first few to be listed, one can conclude that the food, in question, is artificial, and it would be wise to find a more natural alternative. By using this simple technique, it is possible to more judiciously select natural and non-artificial foodstuffs, regardless of where they are purchased.

The practice of reducing or eliminating fake food can drastically increase one's metabolic activity, leading to better overall health. In many traditional health systems, it is often said that good health begins and ends with proper digestion.

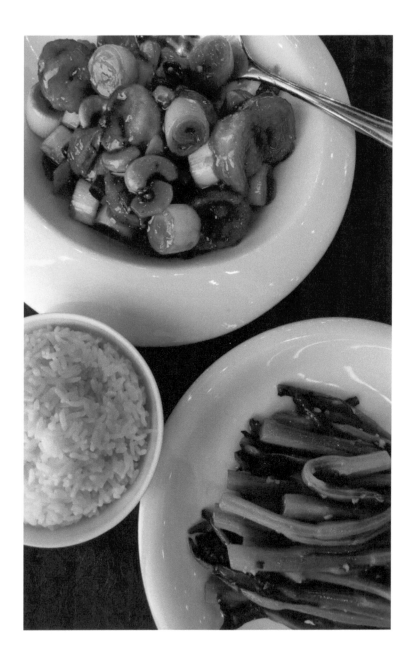

*Dinner: Kung-Pao style prawns with leeks and cashews,
choy sum, and steamed rice*

4 BALANCING NUTRITION

What is "nutrition" and what is "nutritious?" For an ostensibly health-obsessed society, I don't believe that Americans ask these questions enough. Before discussing the topic of balancing nutrition, let us first define the concepts.

From the perspective of Tibetan Medical Science, nutrition is defined as that which sustains the physical body. When saying that something is nutritious, the typical supposition is that such thing is "good for you," or promotes overall health. Although this can be true, it can just as well be false...

In our early 21st century United States, as well as in a host of other developed nations, lifestyle diseases have become an epidemic. Excessively nutritious diets coupled with sedentary lifestyles are causing high incidences of obesity, diabetes, arteriosclerotic diseases, and a host of other illnesses. Therefore, excessively consuming nutritious foods— "excessively" being the operative word—can be bad for one's health. The principle, simply stated, is that too much nutrition can be just as bad, and at times, even worse than too little.

While there is nothing inherently bad about foods high in nutrition, such as bananas, avocados, meats, milk, cheese, or nuts, they can indeed be deleterious to one's health if consumed in excess, and, or, in an imbalanced manner. Hence, the title of this chapter: "Balancing Nutrition."

Having thus defined "nutrition," we must now discuss what is meant by the term "balance." For completeness' sake, let us first reiterate the conclusions reached about proper dietary practices in the previous chapters.

1. **Avoid fake, or non-natural foods.**
   They are technically not "food" but "food-like" products.

2. **Eat natural food in proper portions.**
   The stomach should at no time be filled to more than 3/4 capacity, with 1/4 being solid food, and 2/4 being liquid.

In Tibetan Medical Science, precise balance of a meal or medicinal formula is achieved by way of equating the heating and cooling *characteristics* of that substance.[6] These characteristics are derivatives of the *6 tastes* and *8 powers*.[7] Though an exhaustive discussion of this technique would be much beyond the scope of this brief treatise, a cursory presentation is nonetheless required.

Every food or medicine can be analyzed in terms of overall taste; and each taste can, in turn, be broken down into powers; and each power can be further broken down into characteristics.[8]

---

[6] The 17 characteristics of substances in Tibetan Medical Science are: smooth, heavy, warm, oily, stable, cold, blunt, cool, flexible, fluid, dry, parched, hot, light, sharp, rough, and mobile.

[7] The 6 tastes are: sweet, sour, salty, bitter, hot (spicy), and astringent (woody). The 8 powers are: heavy, oily, cool, blunt, light, rough, hot, and sharp.

[8] Although there are some powers with the same names as characteristics, they are different concepts altogether: powers include characteristics as the latter is a subset of the former.

To illustrate how the concepts of taste, power, and characteristic are related, as well as how substances can be analyzed with them, please consider the following:

Taste Analysis:
A regular slice of cheese pizza with numerous ingredients has the foremost tastes of sweet and salty.

Power Analysis:
The sweet and salty tastes are both *heavy*, and the sweet taste *oily*. The sweet taste is *cool*, and the salty taste *hot*— so they cancel one another out. Furthermore, though the sweet taste is somewhat *blunt*, the more predominant salty taste is *sharp*. Thus, the sweet and salty tastes in the pizza correspond with the *heavy*, *oily*, and *sharp* powers.

Characteristic Analysis:
Finally, the corresponding characteristics would be the same: *heavy*, *oily*, and *sharp*. We would thus consider this food as having "heating" energies, as two of the three characteristics are heating.

Whether a particular food is heating or cooling to the body may also depend on what part of the food is eaten, what toppings or condiments are added, whether it is consumed hot or cold, and other small but important details. A balanced meal or diet will thus balance the heating and cooling energies of the following attributes:

Heating	Cooling
warm	smooth
oily	heavy
dry	cold
hot	blunt
sharp	cool
	flexible
	fluid
	plain
	stable

Table 1.0 : The "rough," "light" and "mobile" characteristics can be directly attributed to the wind humor, and are only slightly cooling; they have thus been purposely omitted from the above categorizations of heating and cooling. [9]

---

[9] See p. 16 of the following Chapter, "Avoiding Food Bans," for a brief description of each of the 3 humors.

All food and medicine, without exception, can adequately be described using the above 17 characteristics. However, the degree to which each characteristic is present in that food or medicine must be ascertained, as all foods contain a certain amount of each characteristic. When identifying a food, medicine, or diet as having any of the above characteristics, what is actually being discussed is the preponderance therein.

Because considering the characteristics of foods listed in the table above may be overly complicated and impractical for the average person looking to consume a healthful, balanced diet, I propose the following:

1. Eat natural *whole foods* in a variety of hues: red, brown, orange, beige, yellow, green, blue, indigo, violet, etc.[10]
2. Consume the variety of tastes:
   sweet, sour, salty, bitter, hot, astringent.
3. Consume various textures of foods:
   rough, smooth, dry, slimy, fuzzy, etc.
4. Eat various qualities of foods:
   cold, hot, raw and cooked.

---

[10] The term "whole foods" simply refers to the entirety of a fruit, vegetable, grain, or meat. The skin of the potato, fish, or apple should be be consumed along with the meat, for example, as there are essential fibers and nutrients in those parts, optimizing the food's nutritive value to the body. Though meats in the West are often sold "skinless and boneless" for marketability, there is an overwhelming amount of scientific data indicating the benefits of bone broth, animal collagen, and "good" fats interspersed throughout the flesh and beneath the skin of the meat. Much the same can be said for full-fat milk, a whole food, versus the popular non-fat or two-percent variety. Although some parts of foods are unpalatable, and even considered poisonous—as in the case of apple seeds—consuming small amounts of them is effectively innocuous. Conversely, pumpkin and squash seeds are much more abundant in quantity in their respective vegetables, and should be consumed, as they are relatively high in protein content. Nature has thus provided the general blueprint for what to consume in our foods: if it's chewable, palatable, and relatively accessible, it is probably safe and beneficial for consumption. Regarding the palatable and accessible parts of foods, removing certain parts, and consuming others only creates inherent imbalance and reduces the overall nutritive effect.

The word "variety" or "various," is the operative word in each of the four guidelines listed above. The concept indicated by these two semantically related terms is at the heart of what it means to consume a balanced diet. Eating a broad spectrum of naturally-occurring hues, tastes, textures, and qualities allows for the individual to receive a wide range of essential vitamins, minerals, nutrients and other substances that the system needs; furthermore, it promotes a healthy microbiome throughout the body and ensures that both heating and cooling energies are equitably featured in the diet. This is crucial to proper nutrition; especially given the modest biodiversity of the appropriately named "Standard American Diet" (S.A.D.) that many of us adhere to.

When redressing an existing imbalance, whether hot or cold, one purposefully favors those tastes, textures, and qualities promoting the attribute (heating or cooling) in deficiency, all while moderating, or even temporarily eliminating those in excess. This principle of re-balancing is the sole aim of diet used therapeutically, regardless of the medical tradition.

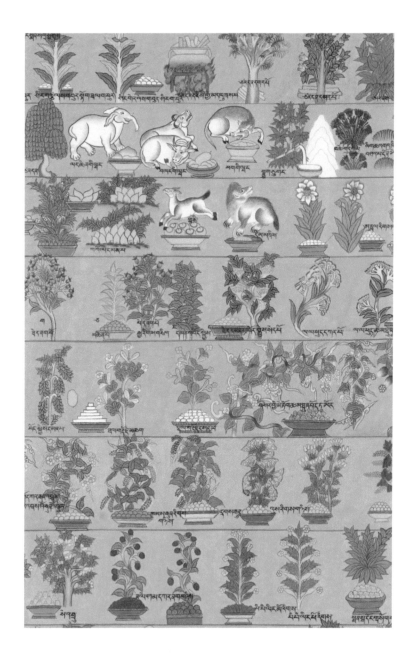

A plate from a Bhutanese collection of the Blue Beryl Thangkas illustrating various types of materia medica

5 AVOIDING FOOD BANS

"Is sugar bad? What about wheat? [...] I try avoiding fats and oils altogether..."

So often, I'm approached with questions and reflections of this kind from people who have gleaned over-simplified dietetic advice from popular daytime talk shows or lifestyle magazines. In this chapter, we will discuss these so-called "food bans" and determine once and for all, what is "healthy" or not!

From the perspective of Tibetan Medical Science, no food is inherently good or bad. While artificial foodstuffs, those with an overwhelming per-weight constitution of artificial ingredients, can be considered categorically bad, a strong argument can be made that they are not even food, but only food-like products.

When discussing real foods, it should be noted that each and every food type has health benefits, as do different types of drinks. The point is not to eliminate any one in particular, but to keep them in balance with one another. To offer the reader some insight into this foundational dietary precept, the following is a brief summary of how various foods and drinks are regarded in the canon of Tibetan Medical Science, as well as some examples of their unique benefits.

First, I will briefly introduce the 3 humors of Tibetan Medical Science: the constitutional building blocks of the human body within this explanatory model. Any discussion of food and drink in Tibetan Medical Science must mention their effect on the body's 3 humors.

The 3 humors are psycho-physical derivatives of the 5 constitutional elements: Earth, Water, Fire, Air, and Space. Air and Space beget the "wind humor," while Fire and Air beget the "bile humor," and Earth and Water, the "phlegm humor."[11] Many other traditional medical systems share similar notions of a humoral theory; while there may be slight differences, this way of viewing the body-mind matrix and connecting it with an environment made up of the same stuff is not unique to Tibetan Medical Science.

The wind humor is invisible and has similar qualities to atmospheric wind: though imperceptible, it is the manifest mover of the leaves fluttering on a tree. Likewise, in the body, it is responsible for all physical and psychological activity; its characteristics are slightly *cool, rough, light,* and *mobile.*[12] Despite being slightly *cool,* wind humor's characteristics are considered neutral, and thus, are neither associated with heating or cooling effects as shown in *Table 1.0.*

The bile humor is that most associated with the heating characteristics of *warm, oily, dry, hot,* and *sharp.* It is similar in nature to the substance found in the gallbladder from which it bears its name, but different in that its scope and functions in the body are more wide-ranging. It is responsible for growth, maturation, metabolism, excretion, and mental acuity, amongst other things.

---

[11] These translations are approximate and cannot be taken as literal equivalents of their English definition—many scholars disagree on just how to translate these scientific medical terms, if at all. For simplicity's sake, I have chosen the terms that are, in my estimation, the closest approximation to the original concepts as presented in the canon of Tibetan Medical Science, "The Secret Tantra of Quintessential Instructions on The Eight Branches of Deathlessness."

[12] Please refer to footnote 6 and Chapter 4, "Balancing Nutrition," for a brief explanation of the 17 characteristics of Tibetan Medical Science.

The phlegm humor is that most associated with the cooling characteristics of *smooth, heavy, cold, blunt, cool, flexible, fluid, plain,* and *stable.* It is also similar in nature to another substance found in the body: mucus; but different in that it's much more expansive in scope and function. Mucus is only one small expression of the energy known as the phlegm humor, which is responsible for firmness and stability of both the mental and physical aspects of being, lubricating the joints, and controlling the body's fluids.

Because both the body and the environment are phenomenological, they share the 5 constitutional elements as building blocks. Given the relationship between the 5 constitutional elements and the 3 humors, as explained above, all food and drink thus increases, decreases, stabilizes or disturbs one, or a combination of the 3 humors throughout the body. Thus, the canon of Tibetan Medical Science categorizes food in 5 types: grains, meats, fats, vegetables, and cooked foods; and explains their effect on the body using the language of these 3 humors and derivative 6 tastes, 8 powers, and 17 characteristics.[13]

Grains are classified into two different categories: awned and leguminous. The awned grains, such as rice, millet, wheat, and barley are sweet in taste, promote virility, pacify the wind humor, and act as a tonic. The leguminous grains, which include peas and beans, are astringent, sweet, and have the characteristics of being *cool, light* and *dry.* Although these grains stop diarrhea and remove grease, they also block the body's channels when consumed in excess. When fresh and wet, grains are heavy in quality; but when ripened, dried, and preserved, they become light. Further cooking by way of boiling or baking makes the grains even lighter and more agreeable for human consumption.

Meats are all considered to be sweet. The flesh of animals living on dry land is *cool, light* and *rough,* and helps bring down certain kinds of fever; whereas the flesh of animals living in wet places is *oily,*

---

[13] Please refer to footnote 6 and 7 for an enumeration of each of the 6 tastes, 8 powers, and 17 characteristics. Fruits are not featured in this classification, perhaps because they are mostly discussed in the various chapters of materia medica.

heavy and *warm* in quality making them effective against disorders of the stomach, kidneys and lower back. The flesh of animals living in both wet and dry areas have some of each of the above qualities. The flesh of birds and carnivorous animals that feed on raw meat has *rough*, *light* and *sharp* qualities. This meat increases the metabolism, promotes healthy weight gain, destroys tumors, and eliminates all disorders classified as being "cold" in nature. Aged meat is especially effective in pacifying wind humor imbalances, and at generating digestive heat.

Fats are of four kinds: butters, seed oils, marrows, and animal fat— they are all sweet in taste. Animal fats are most *heavy* and *cool*, while the various types of butter are the most *light*. Fats help cleanse and lubricate the abdomen: their *blunt*, *subtle*, *smooth* and *moist* characteristics make them ideal for the elderly, infants, and the weak. Fats are also very effective on rough skin and for those deficient in blood and reproductive fluids. Fats can also help calm mental unrest and all disorders associated with the wind humor. Moderate consumption of fats results in healthy metabolism, helping clear internal disorders, good physical strength, radiant complexion, strong sensory organs, and a prolonged life.

Vegetables can either be *warm* and *light* or *cool* and *heavy*, depending on where they were grown and how they are prepared and preserved. Those vegetables having a hot taste, like garlic and onion, or those having a bitter taste, like brussels sprouts and watercress, when collected from dry areas or used in a dried or cooked form, are *warm* and *light*. However, that very same produce, when obtained from wet areas, or used fresh and raw, is *cool* and *heavy*. Onions induce sleep and improve appetite, while garlic helps relieve imbalances of infectious microorganisms like viruses and bacteria. Fresh radishes are *warm* and *light* in quality and support metabolic function; turnips are similar in quality to radishes, though they also protect against all forms of poisoning.

The section on cooked foods includes all of the food categories above. Overall, cooking foods makes them more manageable for the body to digest and assimilate; examples of this are kale, spinach, meats, and most grains. Certain foods, however, are not to be cooked, or only to be cooked lightly. Foods of this kind are easy to masticate and subsequently digest in their natural form, therefore, they need not be cooked to make them easier to consume. Such foods are: cucumbers, melons, and various types of lettuce. Indeed, adding heat to those kinds of foods may make them unpalatable and denature them to the extent that they are no longer nutritionally beneficial for consumption.

How about drinks?

The canon of Tibetan Medical Science describes a variety of drinks and their respective benefits. The text enumerates 7 kinds of water in descending order of superiority: rainwater, snow water, river water, spring water, well water, sea water, and forest water.

Chilled water is beneficial against fainting, exhaustion, hangovers, dizziness, vomiting, thirst, heat, blood disorders, bile humor disorders, and poisoning. Hot boiled water, however, generates body heat and helps with digestion; it instantly relieves hiccups, phlegm humor disorders, stomach distention, asthma, the common cold, and recently contracted communicable diseases. Cooled freshly boiled water is good for bile humor issues, all while not aggravating phlegm humor disorders.

Alcohol is described as generally sweet, sour and bitter, with a sour post-digestive taste.[14] It generates heat, induces courage, increases sleep, and relieves combined phlegm and wind humor disorders. Excessive intake of alcohol, however, is said to yield mental aberration and indiscretion.

Cow's milk is beneficial for many pulmonary disorders, chronic infections, polyuria, mental acuity, and promoting longevity; while goat's milk is particularly beneficial in treating asthma. Sheep's milk is helpful in controlling excess wind humor but is harmful to the

---

[14] Post-digestive tastes are produced by the body after a taste has been metabolized by the numerous digestive functions. The sweet and salty tastes produce the sweet post-digestive taste, while the sour taste remains sour, and the bitter, hot, and astringent tastes produce a bitter post-digestive taste.

heart. Horse and donkey milk strengthen the lungs but also cause mental dullness. Generally, milk that has not been boiled is heavy and cool in quality and can cause microorganic (bacterial and viral) imbalances, as well as phlegm humor disorders. When boiled, it becomes *warm* and *light* and easy to digest. Furthermore, fresh warm milk that has just been milked is like nectar, and has no contraindication.

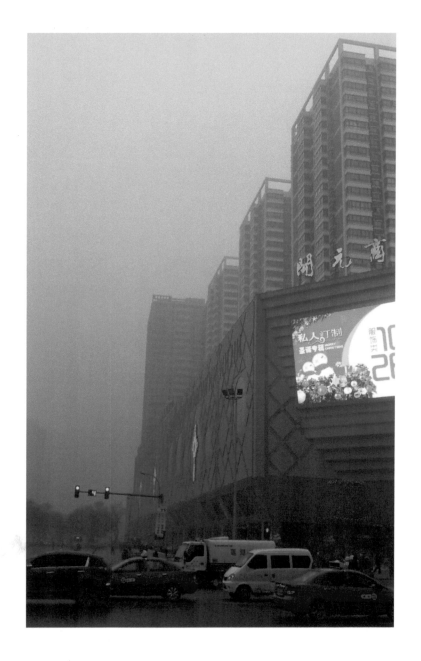

Severe air pollution in Xi'an, Shaanxi Province, P.R.C.

6 REDUCING TOXIC LOAD

The quality of our food and the environment in which this food grows are inextricably linked. Our food all comes from the Earth, though we pollute and abuse its resources. Consequently, the food we eat bears a portion of those same toxins that we introduce into the environment. How then is it possible to consume non-toxic food from a polluted ecosystem? This is a challenge that scientists may not be able to resolve any time soon. Nevertheless, it is indeed possible to take decisive action to reduce our bodies' overall toxic load.

To this end, I propose two solutions:

1. Both individually and collectively minimize pollutants, and encourage the Earth's natural purification processes through sustainable living practices.

2. Patronize natural foods, drinks, medicines, supplements, and cosmetics, for both our own benefit and that of our environment.

While both solutions play into one another, this chapter will more focus on the second.

Minimizing the toxic load in food is one of the most effective means of reducing the body's overall toxic burden. Nowadays, most everyone is aware of the term "organic," as it is prevalent in many grocery stores and frequently mentioned in discussions pertaining to nutrition. The term itself, however, is more of a legal marketing term co-opted by various agencies with fluctuating technical definitions. A brief Google search on the topic will shed more light as to what the precise meaning of the terms "USDA Organic," "Certified Organic," "100% Organic," and others like them are. What's important is that these foods are less adulterated with synthetic chemicals, additives, and other toxic elements that are not germane to our Carbon-based life form. Therefore, when possible, *do buy organic.* While this does not at all guarantee that the product is un-tainted, it will help avoid a large part of the egregiously synthetic elements found in modern-day food products. Furthermore, when buying anything with a food label, it is important to pay attention to what the listed ingredients are, as well as where each ingredient occurs on that list. As previously mentioned in Chapter 3, "Avoiding Fake Food," those ingredients listed foremost are found in highest proportion of the food product.

I. *Reducing the toxic load in our food:*

It is of the utmost importance that consumers learn to read labels—not so much for the caloric content, but for the integrity of ingredients. Many of us purchase food products without scrutinizing the ingredients list and end up regularly consuming such foods. In my experience, the very first thing to look for is one of the prime suspects in adulterated foodstuffs: High Fructose Corn Syrup—the ubiquitous sweetener found in the U.S. and China but banned in European nations. This sweetener is highly toxic to the system due to its wholly synthetic and plasticine nature. From the perspective of Tibetan Medical Science, it is excessively *heavy* and *cool,* effectively clogging the body's channels, and encouraging symptoms similar to those found in obesity: indigestion, chronic fatigue, macular degeneration, upper-respiratory issues, etc. This synthetic compound is used in everything from condiments to breads and pasta sauces. Avoiding this substance and replacing it with real cane sugar, alone, may drastically improve one's health. Though numerous studies have compared High Fructose Corn Syrup to regular naturally-occurring sugar, that is inaccurate and a false equivalency: the former is a sweetener but not a sugar and the latter is a sugar and a sweetener. High Fructose Corn Syrup is in fact not a sugar; it is a purely synthetic compound created for its ease in manufacturing food products at a substantially lower price— there is no reason that one needs this in the diet, and it can be eliminated altogether. In that same way, any other substances that feature prominently in the ingredients list should be scrutinized. Chances are that if one does not recognize the ingredient, it is most likely non-naturally occurring and should be avoided in large doses.

II. *Reducing the toxic load in our drinks:*

To minimize the toxicity in one's drinks, a similar approach to that of food is warranted. It is important, once again, to read the labels on the back of containers, and to avoid any synthetic ingredients as much as possible. Unfortunately, most sweetened drinks in the U.S. also make use of High Fructose Corn Syrup or other artificial sweeteners such as those found in "diet" drinks. These are synthetic sweeteners, which in some measure, poison the system. To be specific, examples of such sweeteners marketed as low-calorie diet substances are aspartame and sucralose. While stevia is a naturally occurring sweetener from a plant, it is also manufactured in non-natural forms. Some stevia-based products even claim to be all natural, though they include dextrose—a refined starch-derived glucose. None of these alternatives are better than natural sugar derived from the sugar cane, or the beet: raw, primary ingredients that grow of the earth and benefit the body, in some measure. In Tibetan Medical Science, naturally derived sugar is considered a medicinal vehicle for all prescriptions formulated to neutralize hot-natured disorders[15]. Therefore, medicines against excesses of the bile humor typically include

---

[15] Please refer to footnote 4 and 5 for more information on what constitutes a "hot-natured" disorder.

natural sugar.

Ultimately, no matter how natural a beverage, it cannot replace the role of pure water in the diet—the most important drink.[16] Per the canon of Tibetan Medical Science, water that has been purified loses this purity after 24 hours. This happens as the liquid gradually leaches elements from its container, and particles in the liquid once filtered out, or broken down by the heat of boiling, start to coalesce anew. Therefore, the common practice of drinking bottled water that has been sitting in a container for long periods of time is less than ideal, especially if said receptacle happens to be made of non-inert, thin, inexpensive plastic. Drinking from freshly boiled or filtered sources can thus greatly reduce the toxic load in our drinking water.

III. *Reducing the toxic load in our medicines:*

Medications can be very toxic to the system when taken in excess of the imbalance that they are intended to redress, or when the side effects are so harsh that they harm the body to an even larger extent than the original disease. For this reason, it is critical for any medical professional to carefully dose prescriptions, especially those that are potent. Failure to do so will ultimately result in the body's detoxification processes being overwhelmed. Even over-the-counter medications designed to be less potent can just as well cause liver issues when taken for an extended period of time. While this in no way is an urging for those with long-term prescriptions to stop taking "necessary" medications, such individuals, or their care takers, should, at the very least, reconsider the treatment plans that they are on.[17] Taking medicines to manage unpleasant

---

[16] Please refer to Chapter 2, "Water Intake," for a more thorough treatment of the importance of consuming pure water.

[17] While the idea of not taking prescription or over-the-counter medications to manage unpleasant symptoms may seem odd, or even reckless, there is a legitimate medical explanation for doing so: managing symptoms without identifying and addressing the root cause can exacerbate a patient's condition, as the principal imbalance goes untreated, and a new imbalance is likely being developed. Should one choose to

symptoms, and more medicines to manage the harsh side effects of the primary prescription, is not a sustainable solution. This eventually leads to chronic maladies, as the cause of the symptomology repeatedly gets swept under the rug. Thankfully, at the time of this writing, there exist a plethora of alternative and complementary medical practices availing holistic health solutions to the Western world, and the world at large—some of which even offer telemedical services. These treatment options can be life-saving, especially for those who have been told that "nothing can be done" regarding their ailment. Irrespective of the healing modality, it should be stated that treating the root cause of an illness in our contemporary medical landscape is possible but rare; as this requires a capable medical professional and a willing patient, both of whom trust in the genuine possibility of complete remediation.[18]

Needless to say, over-consumption of recreational drugs can also leave toxic residues in the system, even when the substance is entirely natural. The idea, again, is that anything in excess, no matter how natural, can cause an imbalance in the body's energies. In an imbalanced system, regular processes of detoxification and elimination are adversely affected, leaving toxins to accumulate in the body.

IV. *Reducing the toxic load in our supplements:*

The supplement industry is a very large and un-regulated international market. From the consumer's perspective, it is incredibly challenging to ascertain what exactly is in the container. Is what the manufacturer purports to be in the bottle actually in the bottle? To the surprise of many, numerous studies have shown regular contamination or, even worse, what seems to be purposeful dissimulation by manufacturers of various supplements. A January 2016 *PBS*

---

cease taking any long-term medications, the canon of Tibetan Medical Science recommends to do so gradually, as to not shock the system.

[18] More on how faith and belief affect healing efficacy in the Conclusion: pp.31-32.

Frontline investigation found that many supplements only contain a small percentage of what is written on the label, if any at all. Furthermore, even when the supplement is entirely unadulterated, how effective is it in helping maintain overall wellness? Is it being properly absorbed by the body? Is the consumer getting too much of it? Are there any contraindications pertaining to that specific consumer that aren't being taken into consideration? There seems to be little to no consensus on the Recommended Daily Allowance (RDA), Adequate Intake (AI), Tolerable Upper Intake Level (UL), or Daily Value (DV) of most nutrients, and the question of "how much is enough?" is complicated by the simple fact that it apparently depends on one's age and gender. What then is a consumer to do? It is the author's belief that it would be best to simply forego taking supplements altogether, and consume a colorful, seasonally-appropriate balanced diet. This not only includes all of the necessary vitamins, minerals, and cofactors needed by the body but also helps maximize absorption of these essential elements in the body.

V. *Reducing the toxic load in our cosmetics:*

Often overlooked for their potentially toxic effects, cosmetics can quickly enter the body through the skin's pores, glands, and superficial vascular channels. Deodorants and antiperspirants with heavy metals and synthetic compounds, as well as lotions, lipsticks, lip balms, soaps, shampoos, conditioners, blush, foundation, eyeliner, and the like, need to be examined for their ingredients, all the same. This is especially true if such products are to be frequently used. Oversight for the cosmetics industry in the U.S. is quite small, though it is a very lucrative market, and an important aspect of the world population's overall toxic load leading to the constellation of diseases found in our societies.

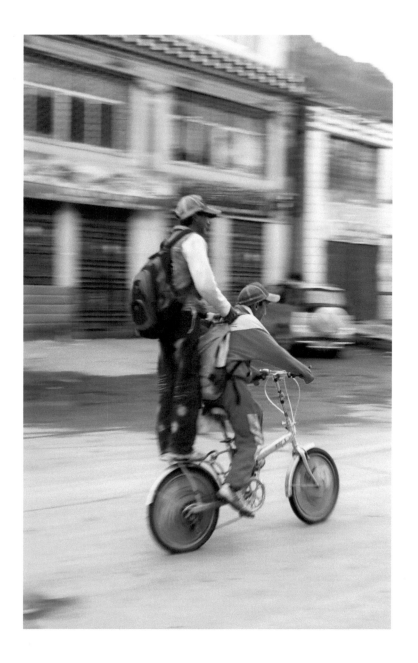

Tibetan boys on their way to school in Yushu, Amdo
Photo Credit: Tsemdo Thar

7 MAINTAINING A NON-SEDENTARY LIFESTYLE

As a preponderance of modern research has shown, a lifestyle with little to no physical activity can prove lethal. Year after year, the so-called "lifestyle diseases" of diabetes and arteriosclerosis are among the leading factors of morbidity and mortality in the U.S., the incidence of which have been shown to be correlated with low levels of physical activity. Although Diet is first and foremost in importance and effectiveness in treating and maintaining proper psycho-physiological health in Tibetan Medical Science, Lifestyle, encompassing regular physical activity, is a close second.[19] Consequently, a lifestyle with moderate exercise is indispensable for the appropriate maintenance of the mind-body complex.

In our modern American culture, there is the prevailing notion that some exercise is good and more is even better—but that isn't always true. Tibetan Medical Science states that walking is the "king" of all exercises, as it can be done by the very young, the old, and everyone in between, with great benefit, and little to no deleterious effect. That last point is crucial. While any form of exercise can greatly benefit its practitioner if properly performed, the opposite can lead to serious injury. The adverse effects of an

---

[19] Please refer to the 4 levels of therapy in Tibetan Medical Science: Diet, Lifestyle, Medicine, Accessory Therapy, as outlined in the Introduction on pp. ii-v.

overly intense exercise regimen, or one done incorrectly without adequate recovery, are biophysical ailments such as sprains, strains, tears, and breaks. Furthermore, Tibetan Medical Science asserts that extreme Lifestyle activities can also produce blockages, excesses, or deficiencies in the wind humor energy throughout the body. These imbalances can gradually destabilize a person's psychology, as one of the major roles of the wind humor is to govern the movement of thoughts and awareness. The wind humor is the link between mind and body; the psychological and the physiological; this has yet to be discovered in Western biomedicine.[20] Thus, physical trauma can yield psychological trauma even when injury to the brain has not been sustained (as in Chronic Traumatic Encephelopathy), or when such physical trauma is not coupled with an emotionally destabilizing event.

In sum, moderate exercise is paramount to the maintenance and re-establishment of proper psycho-physiological health. Care must be taken so that the activity, whatever it may be, is performed with proper technique and in proper measure.

What specific exercise should I be doing?

It shouldn't matter as long as the activities include the following three aspects: stretching, deep breathing, and resistance. Each one of these features is necessary for adequate maintenance of the body—namely for those of us who sit for long periods of time during a typical day, engage in limited repetitive motions, or are otherwise largely inactive. Although walking has been highlighted for reasons previously mentioned, examples of other comprehensive exercises are: running, martial arts, swimming, hatha yoga, gymnastics, and various kinds of dancing...to name a few

---

[20] See p. 16 of Chapter 5, "Avoiding Food Bans," for a brief description of the wind humor.

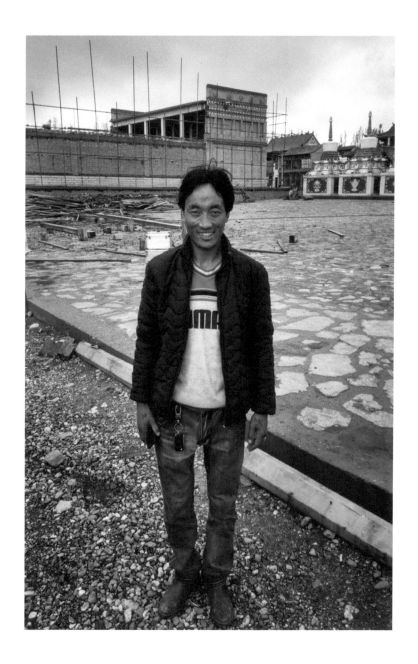

A friend of the author smiling at a monastery in Amdo

8 CHOOSING A POSITIVE PERSPECTIVE

The idea of choosing a positive perspective is often cited as a general piece of good advice, though it is seldom explained. What does it mean, and how can it be of benefit? While modern psychology and neuroscience have begun to address some of these questions in the context of neurotransmitters and reward centers, Tibetan Medical Science's holistic explanatory model offers a different perspective.

As outlined in Chapter 5, "Avoiding Food Bans," the 3 humors of Tibetan Medical Science, loosely translated as the wind humor, the bile humor, and the phlegm humor, serve as the constitutional building blocks of the human body. These 3 humors are a byproduct of our consciousness, arising at conception from psychopathological afflictions in our karmic imprint, or soul memory. Experiences in feeling desirous attachment are said to generate the wind humor; while feelings of anger and hatred generate the bile humor; and feelings of mental obtuseness generate the phlegm humor. Mental obtuseness, in this sense, relates to not paying attention to oneself, and dulling the senses through perpetual distraction, such as in the mindless consumption of sensory stimuli to fill an emotional void.[21] Nevertheless,

---

[21] It is not uncommon for many of us to bombard our external senses with stimuli: from mindlessly watching television and reviewing our social media threads only a few moments after putting our devices down, eating

according to Tibetan Medical Science, without the karmic imprint of the aforementioned negative feelings, we do not create the 3 humors, which actually allow us to form this psycho-physiological ego to experience phenomenological existence. Thus, the favorable opportunity for a rare and precious human life presents itself, in part, due to these negative perceptions.

Having now established the link between the 3 humors of wind, bile, and phlegm, as well as the perceptions of desirous attachment, hatred, and mental obtuseness, it is possible to comprehend how negative perspectives can affect one's entire being by modulating one's constitutional humors out of balance. Specifically, desirous attachment of any kind increases and disturbs the wind humor, while hatred and anger increase and disrupt the bile humor, and mental obtuseness increases and disrupts the phlegm humor. Given that these humors make up the entire psycho-physiological body, it is essential for proper functioning of the system that they are all well balanced and in appropriate measure. The disruption of these humors by negative perceptions thus adversely affects an individual's entire mind-body complex. Conversely, when a person manages to do away with these original faults of perception, i.e. completely do away with attachment, hatred and mental obtuseness, the old patterns are broken, and the individual is said to have ascended the very etiology of all disease. Simply put, persistently keeping negative perceptions at bay may allow for one to escape the very quagmire of disease itself! Having thus removed these psychological precursors to the quasi-physical 3 humors, one theoretically no longer creates the humors, making it such that there is no longer anything left to balance or disrupt. Keeping a positive perspective to the point of eliminating one's constitutional humors, is thus the ultimate medicine and lifelong achievement.

---

to cope with an emotional void, or engaging in sexual activity to fulfill the same. Such behavior actively diverts our attention from the introspection necessary to address those feelings of inadequacy, as we continue to do anything but confront our internal challenges.

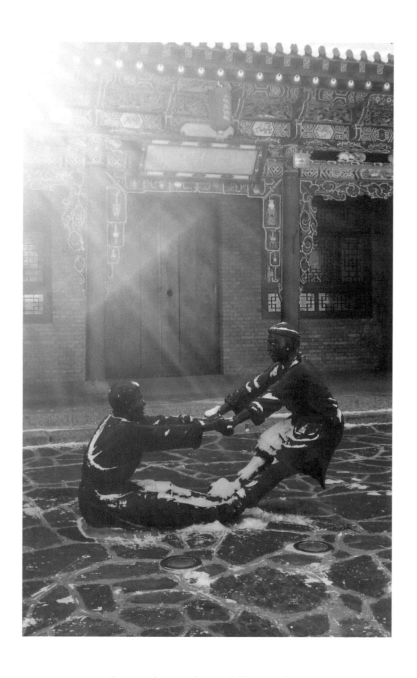

A statue depicting happy children at play—
seemingly free from the anxieties plaguing most of their adult counterparts

CONCLUSION

Health is freedom: freedom to apply the faculties of the mind and body as one sees fit; freedom to take in the occasional unbalanced meal; freedom to live in a moderately polluted environment, drink slightly contaminated water, and breathe dirty city air, yet still manage to expel wastes and avoid a morbid existence. All of this is why health is invaluable. Health is also a choice: in so far as many—though not all—health issues, are a direct or indirect result of our choosing to eat and live in non-healthful ways.

Because the path from health to disease is usually a choice (though not always a conscious one), the path back from disease to health is as well. This is not only limited to choosing to see a doctor, a therapist, or any other health professional for guidance on how to re-establish health but, more importantly, it involves following through with the necessary dietetic and lifestyle recommendations, which invariably accompany any complete treatment plan. As stated in multiple instances throughout this treatise, Diet and Lifestyle are of chief importance in most any treatment plan, and the "patient" controls whether or not the plan is properly executed. In truth, the patient is the real doctor, and the doctor or health professional is more like a coach, guiding said patient on how to properly eat, live, and on whether or not to take medicines or undergo any accessory therapies.

No matter the system, medical tradition, or title of the health professional, it is up to the patient, the recipient of the treatment plan, to properly execute the treatment as thoroughly as possible. More importantly, it is necessary that the patient trust in the possibility, the chance, that their chosen health professional and his or her treatment plan is well capable of achieving the desired prognosis. This cannot be overstated. In Western allopathic medicine, this effect is relegated to what is called "placebo," which, at this point, is mostly a catch-all for inexplicable non-physical therapeutic outcomes. Rather, in Tibetan Medical Science, and many other traditional health disciplines, this concept is fairly well understood. For healing to take place, on some level of consciousness, the patient is required to co-create the experience of wellness with the healer. Meaning, the patient must first believe in the possibility of healing being achieved with the aid of that particular healer or healing modality, then, on the basis of that belief, the patient is able to create the experience of having been healed. Without this, it is very challenging to reverse any disorder, especially those of a deep-seated nature. This can explain what happens in "faith healings" or other healings of seemingly miraculous nature where no ostensible therapeutic technique has been applied. Therefore, it is fitting that patients who are averse to a particular healing modality, or lend very little credence to that system, will experience relatively low rates of therapeutic success; conversely, those who hold a particular system in high regard, or who view a particular healer in the same manner, will experience relatively high rates of therapeutic success. The canon of Tibetan Medical Science clearly describes how one of the roles of the physician-healer is to inspire confidence in all of his or her patients, in part, through a good reputation, and continuous positive reinforcement. Thus, according to Tibetan Medical Science, patients with a positive outlook, even on a bleak prognosis, give themselves a much better chance to achieve their desired wellness goals.

I hope that the Eight Principles shared in this treatise are understood as being timeless and universally applicable, regardless of which medical tradition one espouses. Despite these Principles being couched in the language and theory of Tibetan Medical Science, a relatively ancient medical tradition, they should be recognized as being germane to our human body and our phenomenological universe. Whether you are a patient, a health professional, or just a casual reader: may these principles further elucidate and facilitate your quest for achieving health.

ABOUT THE AUTHOR

EzDean Fassassi was born in Washington D.C. to immigrant parents from West Africa. After graduating from Princeton University in 2007 and spending a year developing vaccines at Children's Hospital of Philadelphia, he discovered Tibetan Medicine while scouring the Medical Anthropology section at UPenn's Van Pelt Library. From there, he studied the ancient medical system with Tibetan physicians in exile in Western Massachusetts, then in Western China. While living in Qinghai Province, he wrote the first edition of The Tibetan Phrasebook (2013) and completed his practicum under the guidance of accomplished physicians. In late 2014 he opened Holistic Health Consulting, an appointment-only clinic located in the Washington D.C. metropolitan area, where he's practiced Tibetan Medical Science ever since.

CPSIA information can be obtained
at www.ICGtesting.com
Printed in the USA
BVHW051943141219
566538BV00004B/7/P

* 9 7 8 1 7 3 2 5 8 4 9 3 8 *